YOUR KNOWLEDGE HAS VALUE

- We will publish your bachelor's and master's thesis, essays and papers

- Your own eBook and book - sold worldwide in all relevant shops

- Earn money with each sale

Upload your text at www.GRIN.com and publish for free

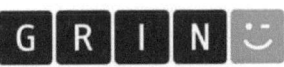

Jochen Schmidt

Ambulance Response Times in Developing Emergency Health Care Systems

GRIN Publishing

Bibliographic information published by the German National Library:

The German National Library lists this publication in the National Bibliography; detailed bibliographic data are available on the Internet at http://dnb.dnb.de .

Imprint:

Copyright © 2006 GRIN Verlag GmbH
Print and binding: Books on Demand GmbH, Norderstedt Germany
ISBN: 978-3-640-34746-9

This book at GRIN:

http://www.grin.com/en/e-book/129060/ambulance-response-times-in-developing-emergency-health-care-systems

GRIN - Your knowledge has value

Since its foundation in 1998, GRIN has specialized in publishing academic texts by students, college teachers and other academics as e-book and printed book. The website www.grin.com is an ideal platform for presenting term papers, final papers, scientific essays, dissertations and specialist books.

Visit us on the internet:

http://www.grin.com/

http://www.facebook.com/grincom

http://www.twitter.com/grin_com

Ambulance Response Times in Developing Emergency Health Care Systems

by

Jochen Schmidt

EMS 450 Baccalaureate Capstone Project

Andrew Jackson University, Birmingham, Alabama, USA

03.09.2006

Ambulance Response Times in Developing Emergency Health Care Systems

Outline

Thesis: Dispatcher training can improve ambulance response times in EMS systems in low income countries.

I.   Statement of the problem

    A. Introduction

        1. Why was the research started

        2. We need to improve health care in 3rd world countries.

        3. In order to do this, we need to improve emergency care.

            A. Why emergency care?

            B. Why focus on this?

            C. Ambulance response time plays an important role in improving the outcome of patients in health emergencies.

        4. Ambulance response time has impact on short-term survival.

        5. Need for sustainable approaches in low- and middle- income countries in order to improve emergency health care. One approach could be ambulance response time.

II.   Survey of the literature

    A. How do we improve emergency care in an area with limited resources?

    B. Training is one way to do this.

    C. Dispatcher Training can be effective.

        1. What training programs are available for dispatchers?

    D. How do we evaluate the effectiveness of our training?

        1. Look at ambulance response times

a. Is this a good method?

    i. Some say yes – why?

        1. Ambulance response has been area of interest in recent years.

        2. Ambulance response is prone to perceptions, demands and utilization of emergency medical services.

        3. Changes are necessary in order to improve response time.

        4. Example of changes from Canada.

        5. Study that changes in developing countries should focus on ambulance response. Support of pilot projects and research.

    ii. Some say no – why?

        1. Arguments against focus on ambulance response time.

        2. Widespread development of indicators is needed.

        3. No universal approach to emergency medical service performance indicators has been developed so far.

        4. Traditional approach to performance measurement should be questioned.

     5. The right development of indicators is

       questioned.

    b. Counter argument

      1. Example of Addis Ababa shows that a case sensitive

        assessment of performance indicators and focus of

        change should be developed – in individual case can

        this be ambulance response time.

III.   Research design and data collection

   A. Study design and protocol:

     i. Experimental research design

     ii. Collect data for ambulance response times before and after implementation

       of training program

   B. Subjects

     i. Osh Ambulance description

     ii. Dispatchers in that system – description and level of education

     iii. Ambulance workers - description

   C. Interventions

     i. Training program – description

     ii. Tone system - description

   D. Measurements and other observations

   E. Explanation of results and relation to examples from the literature.

V. Conclusion

   A. Result supports thesis and importance of topic.

   B. Further research in this area is needed.

Ambulance Response Times in Developing Emergency Health Care Systems

Abstract

Dispatcher training can improve ambulance response times in emergency medical service (EMS) systems in low income countries. Emergency health care systems are of increasing concern in international healthcare developments and the global fight against the burdens of disease. Studies show that emergency health care improvements in developing countries should focus on ambulance response. Low-cost changes including emergency medical dispatch training in developing urban emergency health care systems can improve ambulance response times. Concerns about focusing on ambulance response time as a single indicator are addressed by showing a case sensitive approach for developing emergency health care systems that in return can identify ambulance response as main indicator for a particular system. This approach has been chosen for the subject of study, the Osh Ambulance Service, a municipal EMS in Kyrgyzstan. This particular service, the implemented research, the study design and, the data analysis are presented. The data show that there has been a change from an average response time of 23, 18 minutes to 20, 15 minutes. This data is statistically significant and indicates that the implemented changes, despite severe challenges, likely have an effect, but it is unclear if this change will have a large clinical impact. Further research on emergency medical dispatch and emergency medical response in low- and middle- income countries is encouraged. With increased opportunities and further globalization emergency health care professionals could play a greater role in research and development of emergency medical service systems in resource-limited countries.

Ambulance Response Times in Developing Emergency Health Care Systems

1. Statement of the problem

This research was based on the experience of the authors in emergency medical service (EMS) development and training in low-income countries. As one would expect, the problems with ambulance response are many and varied. They range from poor road conditions, lack of equipment and vehicles, overspecialization of the ambulance units, lack of training for dispatchers, frequent power outages which limit the radio usage and a limited supply of gasoline for the ambulances themselves. When thinking about what vast resources are necessary to address the complex web of problems, the question surfaced; if dispatcher training can improve ambulance response times in low income countries?

Health care systems in low- and middle income countries need improvement and support in order to ease the global burden of disease and enable human development. A lot of financial resources are poring into third world countries in order to accomplish this.

Emergency health care is becoming an important focus in international health care development. Emergency medical services are seen as a critical component of health care in developing countries (Kobusingye, 2005). It has been recognized as an important horizontal approach to improve living conditions, burdens of disease and long-lasting economic effects due to improved disease adjusted life years (DALYs) in industrialized nations and developing countries alike (Davis, 2004; Kellermann, 2002). Rather than focusing on a vertical (disease oriented) approach a horizontal approach like on emergency medical services provides benefits to the population suffering from various medical conditions.

If we define EMS systems based on experiences from industrialized nations system development and improvements will fail in the Third World because resources in low- and middle- income countries (LIMC) are limited and sustainable approaches are needed in order to develop an emergency health care system with a lasting effect for the population (Kobusingye, 2005).

Changes need to be made that are able to be maintained by the health care system long after international aid has vanished. Otherwise there are a lot of resources and time that is wasted. Indeed many people in third world countries still do not have access to proper emergency care and equipment. This results from a lack of infrastructure and financial resources (Jamison 2006; Kobusingye 2005).

2. Survey of the literature

How can we improve emergency care in a region with limited resources and maintain a sustainable approach? Before changes are implemented and further investments are made into the area of emergency medical services in developing countries it is important to find support for this approach. Hauswald and Yeoh (1997) have studied this issue and came to the conclusion that the benefits of an EMS system for a developing country are small if it is based on western models. The authors support the search for alternative approaches to a North American EMS model in low- and middle-income countries. Also Kobusingye (2005) concludes that EMS system development must be carefully designed to the countries needs.

Practice and research in emergency health care and in particular in ambulance services have focused in the last 30 to 40 years on health care system in developed and industrialized nations. The focus of research often was to improve emergency health care delivery in these regions. How important are emergency medical services for developing countries, and how important is the improvement of ambulance response for low- and middle- income countries? These questions need to be asked in the light of low levels of infrastructure, health care services, income and education in these regions – factors that influence ambulance response and the overall performance of emergency health care systems.

In 1995 a comparative study of Ghana and Mexico (Arreola-Risa) found out that in order to improve trauma care (as part of emergency health care) in urban areas of developing countries the focus should be on ambulance service and emergency room development rather than on intensive care unit development and other levels and areas of care.

Razzak and Kellermann (2002) support research and pilot projects in the area of emergency health care development in low and middle income countries. They show that the incorporation of a basic level of emergency medical care into a health system ha a significant impact on the well-being of the populations.

This view is also shared by a recent publications of the World Bank: "Disease Control Priorities in Developing Countries – 2nd Edition" provides data that shows that 36% of all disability adjusted life years (DALYs) in low- and middle- income countries could benefit from emergency medical service systems if they would be available (Jamison (Ed.), 2006).

In resource limited settings it is important to determine what kind of changes can possibly have a positive impact on emergency medical service performance. The authors of a case study on developing countries found the following: "Prevention, as well as improvements in prehospital care are likely priorities for developing countries" (Mock, 2003, p.45). The paper identifies three different categories that should be addressed: Administration and organization, human resources including staffing and training, physical resources like equipment, supplies and infrastructure. The authors show that improvements in organizational measures like the introduction of improved dispatch schemes can have an impact in the essential health service delivery of emergency care.

Strengthening organizational means are a method how an EMS system can be influenced. One way to influence such organizational capacities is training, and a crucial point in ambulance response is the mechanism of ambulance dispatch. Therefore a dispatch training program likely can influence the process of ambulance dispatch. As a consequence this paper asks if dispatcher training can improve ambulance response times in EMS systems in low income countries.

What kinds of training programs are available for emergency medical service dispatchers? The most widespread used training program is the emergency medical dispatch curriculum of the National Highway Traffic Safety Administration (Wallace (Ed.), 1995). This program has been adopted by many emergency medical service systems and changed to their specific needs. Currently dispatch training based on this program is not only performed in the USA, it serves as a template and emergency medical dispatch programs in Germany, the UK, as well as other countries are based on this curriculum.

In an attempt to evaluate the effectiveness of dispatch training ambulance response times can serve as an indicator. Ambulance response times play an important role in improving the outcome of patients in health emergencies (Pell, 2001). Response times and response time regulation is therefore a topic that not only affects developing emergency health care systems but also systems that are already firmly in place.

Is ambulance response time a good indicator for EMS system performance? Ambulance response time has often been an area of interest with those concerned with the development of emergency health care systems. A paper by Kellermann & Razzak shows that improved ambulance times in developing countries can limit mortality and morbidity, and have a positive impact on injury complication, infection and early rehabilitation of sick and injured patients (2002). Mayer (1979) shows that ambulance response times have an impact on short-term survival and that ambulance response is influenced by the patients delay to seek care, by dispatch time and the ambulance travel time to the scene of the emergency. Especially the dispatch time and the ambulance travel time are factors that can be influenced through organizational means.

The Irish Association of Ambulance Personnel claims that as many as 700 people die each year because of long ambulance response times in rural areas (Payne, 2000). It can take up to 20 minutes to dispatch an ambulance after a call in these places. This poor response time is due to lack of funding and organizational errors within the Irish EMS systems. All problems are not solved by training alone, and are not limited to the developing world.

In specific emergency cases, this response time is often perceived as taking longer than it actually does (which would make sense from a psychological point of view), however the public's general perception of the timeliness of EMS response plays an important role in the utilization of such a system (Finch, 1999). This demonstrates that the public is interested in improved response times and the picture the ambulance service portrays also influences its utilization and therefore its capability to respond in time at the event of a health emergency.

The question that needs to be asked is what is the most efficient use of resources to make change regarding emergency medical service delivery. Stiell and colleagues (1999) have shown that low cost improvements in a Canadian emergency medical service system can have a positive impact on ambulance response times. His paper shows that a multifaceted optimization approach focusing on improving the dispatch process, and continuous quality improvement can lead to significant improvements in survival rates in a large Basic Life Support (BLS) and defibrillation based emergency medical service system. Stiell, et al shows that low cost improvements can have an effect on response times. In this particular study the 8 minute response goal has improved from 76.7 % times of all calls before changes got introduced to 92, 5 % after changes were in place.

A similar study was conducted in the city of Monterrey in Mexico also focusing on low cost changes. The data from this study was published in 2000. In this study focusing on the emergency medical service system in Monterrey the response time decreased from a mean of 15, 5 minutes while there where two dispatch sites to 9, 5 minutes when there where four dispatch sites. The increase in sites of dispatch and other low cost measurements (in this case it was prehospital trauma life support training) resulted in improved response times and lower mortality rates. The authors conclude that the changes where low cost and should be considered for use in other developing countries. This study emphasizes the point that low-cost changes can have a positive impact on health care delivery and outcome (Arreola-Risa, 2000).

Short ambulance times are important, but a goal of a 5-minute response time for acute cases is not realistic in a low- income country. Pell (2001) from the UK states that an ambulance response time of 5 minutes could almost double the survival rate for unwitnessed cardiac arrest. This 5 minute response time needs a very well developed infrastructure. With the limited resources available in low income countries such an effort would not be sustainable. Resources should be spent on a sustainable response system as well as on improvements in facility based emergency health care.

There are many voices that question the use of ambulance response time as a performance indicator. O'Meara (2005) in his paper expresses concern about focusing solely on response times as an indicator of good emergency response. He asks that there would be a widespread development of other indicators for ambulance service delivery. More concerns are expressed by Moore (1999). Moore asked if evaluation and research of emergency medical service systems has any importance as long as there are no universally accepted systems or approaches for evaluation of emergency medical services. The author particularly questions traditional approaches and recognizes the diverse circumstances under which emergency medical services operate. Farlane (2003) emphasizes in his work the difficulty that occurs when evaluating and comparing ambulance service systems. They ask if global indicators could be developed and if the right indicators have been developed.

Some papers show that a single focus on a simple indicator like ambulance response time might not correctly evaluate an emergency health care system but yet despite these concerns there still needs to be a way to evaluate an EMS system. A study on the EMS system of the city of Addis Ababa in Ethiopia concludes that the capacities for EMS need to be assessed in every single situation in order to prioritize needs and develop a sustainable concept for improvement (Pozner, 2003). It is shown that in each case with a focus on a particular system the ambulance response time can be the main indicator and focus of change in order to improve the overall system performance. This approach was chosen in the particular case of the ambulance service in Osh, Kyrgyz Republic.

3. Research design and data collection

A prospective observational study with an experimental design was designed to compare ambulance response times before and after the implementation of an ambulance dispatch training program.

As an example of a developing emergency health care system and subject of study, the ambulance service of the city of Osh in the Kyrgyz Republic was chosen. In the 1960s health authorities of the Soviet Union (USSR) developed ambulance service systems to serve the population in need of urgent health care. Since the collapse of the USSR, due to political and economic changes these systems are under jeopardy. The Kyrgyz ambulance service system is very similar to the Russian model (Townes, 1998) and to models that exist in other Central Asian countries (Partridge, 1998). Due to the economic crisis of the country, health care authorities try to control health care expenses in creating synergies. In 2003 the Ministry of Health decided to hand over the responsibility for ambulance service from the district hospitals to the newly created family medical centers (Meimanaliev, 2005). This was done in order to group competencies in prehospital care.

The Osh Ambulance Service is a municipal service that is funded through two sources: a republican budget and mandatory health insurance organization. In this regard the ambulance service is one of the few exceptions because the ambulance service is independent from the family medical center structures and receives funds from two budgets. Osh is the second largest city in the Kyrgyz Republic and the capital of Osh region as well as the economic center of Southern Kyrgyzstan.

The service has 10 ambulance vehicles available to respond to emergencies. The dispatch center can be reached by dialing 103 (a number similar to 911 in the US or 112 in Europe). All ambulances as well as the dispatch center utilize FM-radio equipment. The service responds to emergencies within an urban area with an estimated population 450 000. 6 ambulance crews consist of a driver, one feldsher (health care practitioner with a 3 year education) and a physician. 4 ambulance teams consist of a feldsher and one ambulance driver. Some ambulance teams are specialized in order to respond to psychiatric, pediatric, and cardiac emergencies.

The ambulance service in Osh, like in many other low- and middle- income countries is suffering from several factors that influence ambulance response time that are difficult to control. Equipment, supplies, fuel and overall funds are limited. Frequently ambulances are taken out of service for maintenance, patients are asked to provide money for fuel, and power cuts limit the use of the radio system (Shepard, 1999). Some ambulances lack warning lights & siren, road conditions are far from acceptable, and phone connections are frequently interrupted.

Besides these there are other factors that can be controlled by the ambulance service management. These are especially human factors (training) as well as organizational means. Until the implementation of changes mentioned in this paper there has been no formal and systematic means that would enable ambulance dispatch to differentiate between urgent or non-urgent calls within the activation process for ambulance crews. Because of this fact almost all ambulance calls were handled in a non-urgent manner.

The ambulance service employs several categories of ambulance workers:
1. Drivers: Drivers have a short training course in vehicle maintenance and some drivers have a 5-day first aid training course, others are trained on the job by mid-level medical personnel.
2. Sanitaries: Sanitaries are medical orderlies with no training. They often work in cleaning ambulance vehicles as well as maintaining the ambulance station. They also support other personnel in their duties at the station.
3. Feldshers: A feldsher is a mid-level health care provider who can perform several medical procedures independently. They graduate from a 3 year vocational college. Some feldshers have a specialized training as feldsher anesthetist. This training has no specific focus on Prehospital emergency care.
4. Doctors: Doctors work as specialized ambulance physicians (cardiology, pediatric, resuscitation, internal medicine) and work on specialized ambulances as well as non-specialized

ambulances. Doctors work also as supervisors at the ambulance station. Emergency Medicine is not recognized as a specialty or subspecialty in Kyrgyzstan.

All dispatchers have an education as feldsher and are supervised by a physician supervisor who overseas the daily work of the dispatch staff, the road ambulance teams and a small first aid post which is attached to the ambulance station. The dispatchers decide on the nature of the call (preliminary diagnosis) if the patient only receives advice by phone or if an ambulance is needed to see the patient.

Most of the staff (except for ambulance drivers) has received basic training in prehospital emergency care (2-4 weeks) through training programs developed with the support of international donor organizations. A limited number of mid-level and physician personnel have participated in a pilot three-month Prehospital emergency care qualification. In Osh 50% of all drivers and sanitaries have participated in a 5-day First Responder training based on the USDOT training curriculum.

The Osh Ambulance Service and the Osh Emergency Medical Service Training Center (a department of the Kyrgyz State Medical Institute for Postgraduate Training and Continuous Education) agreed on a research design as shown in table-1. The elements of this research design include the introduction of dispatch training and implementation of low cost changes and an assessment of improvement.

Ambulance response time data as well as preliminary diagnostic data were collected before and after the implementation of emergency medical dispatch training and associated low-cost technical changes. Ambulance response time was measured on a standard, calibrated clock starting with the activation of the emergency medical service system (caller calls 103 number) and ending with the arrival of the ambulance team at the scene of the emergency.

For the actual measurement of response times only urgent calls were considered. All participating institutions where informed about the research project and data collection sheets were designed in order to record the data. For the actual data collection process a research assistant with a good command of the English language was hired. The research assistant was trained on how to use the data collection sheets and about her role as an observer/research assistant at the Osh Ambulance Dispatch Center.

In early May 2006 on 6 subsequent days during a daily period of 7 hours data including: call time, ambulance dispatch time, ambulance arrival time and preliminary diagnosis were recorded on especially developed forms. On 3 days data collection was performed in the morning hours from 8:30 am to 4:30 pm. On 3 days data collection was performed in the evening hours from 1:00 pm to 9:00 pm.

After this 6 day period all dispatchers of the Osh Ambulance Service received a 40-hour emergency medical dispatch training (DPS = dispestherski plan skoraja i neotloshnaja medizinski pomosh). The curriculum is based on the Emergency Medical Dispatch Course of the US Department of Transportation (Wallace (Ed.), 1995) and has been modified slightly and translated into Russian in order to meet the differences in culture, language, organization as well as the availability of specific emergency services and infrastructure in urban areas of the Kyrgyz Republic. The training consisted of giving written materials, showing interactive presentations, and teaching practical lessons which included critical situations and mock patient calls. The training program was repeated throughout the month of May 2006 in order to train all ambulance dispatchers employed with the Osh Ambulance Service.

All ambulance supervisors received written material and a text in order to familiarize themselves with the DPS-program. All ambulance teams received an informal training on the

DPS-program. All ambulances and dispatch places were equipped with DPS-charts that were intended to assist the ambulance service during the ambulance response process.

During the same period of time a radio engineer has implemented several changes. All rooms of the ambulance station were equipped with an audio/visual – system in order to activate ambulance crews for urgent calls (Table-2). The FM radio system was changed in order to send an audio signal that would alert ambulance teams about an urgent call.

After the implementation and testing of this new system a second week of data collection followed in June 2006. On 6 subsequent days of one week during a daily period of 7 hours data was collected. On 3 days data collection was performed in the morning hours from 8:30 am to 4:30 pm. On 3 days data collection was performed in the evening hours from 1:00 pm to 9:00 pm. During both weeks the same data collection sheets were utilized and the same research assistant performed the data collection. The data was recorded in excel spread sheet, and a student's t-test was performed.

4. Results

There were a total of 923 calls recorded. The call record data and number is located in Table-3. Of these calls, they were classified as to acute or urgent calls and non-urgent calls based on the preliminary data that was recorded. Prior to the intervention, during the first week, 51% of the calls were classified as urgent calls and post intervention, during the second week; approximately 60% of the total calls were classified as acute or urgent calls. This data is located in Table-4, along with a further analysis of the non- urgent calls. Only the acute or urgent calls were analyzed for ambulance response time. Before implementation of the dispatch training, the average ambulance response time was 23.2 minutes with a standard deviation of 17.8 minutes

(Table-6). The average ambulance response time after implementing the program at the Osh Ambulance Service was calculated to be as 20.2 minutes; with a standard deviation is 18.4 minutes. This results in a difference of 3, 03 minutes. (P value is <=0.033)This result is statistically significant if an error rate of 5% (α) is calculated. The attached graph visualizes these results (Graph-1). The acute calls also were analyzed as to type. This result is located in Table-5. Noteworthy is the low category of trauma calls (5% or less). The cardiac calls were 29.9% and 31.1 % respectively. These calls included hypertension and hypertensive crisis as well as "cardiac" category.

5. Discussion

It is likely that the implemented changes have had an effect on the ambulance response time. The statistical significance however is contrasted with clinical health care outcomes. It has to be assumed that only a few patients will benefit from the improved ambulance response time as the average response time is still very high above the recommendation of 4-6 minutes (McSwain, 1991) or of 8 minutes within the Canadian OPALS study (Stiell, 1999).

Mc Swain has based his findings on the number of one ambulance team per population of 50,000. The Osh Ambulance Service assuming that all vehicles are available and running has one ambulance team per 45,000. In Monterrey, Mexico the average response time is 10 minutes while there is one ambulance team serving a population of 100,000 (Kobusingye, 2005). In Hanoi, Vietnam the average ambulance response time is 30 minutes with only one ambulance team serving a population of 600,000 (Mock, 1998).

There are many reasons within the Osh emergency health care system that can be the cause for a response time of 20 minutes with a ratio of ambulance per population of 1:45 000. There are only two dispatch places available. An increase of dispatch sites and phone lines, like in Monterrey, Mexico might improve dispatch response time. In Monterrey the response time was improved from an average of 15, 5 minutes to 9, 5 minutes by establishing two additional dispatch sites (Arreola-Risa, 2000). Another reason for a relatively slow response could be that ambulances are stationed only at one single ambulance station. In the last 15 years existing satellite stations have been closed due to financial restrictions.

Other reasons that based on poor infrastructure and significant financial restrictions can also result in significant delay in response. Fuel limitations, old and fragile ambulance vehicles, as well as interrupted phone lines and cultural restrictions might also contribute to these delays.

Misplaced calls are all calls where the caller picked the wrong phone number, or the phone line got disconnected, or the call was an attempted joke. Private calls are calls were people wanted to talk to ambulance service staff in a private matter. In many EMS systems many of the misplaced and private calls would be categorized as an abuse of the emergency number. In Kyrgyzstan a poor telecommunications infrastructure often does not leave many choices for persons than to use the emergency number in order to access information and contact with people. The situation is rather suboptimal and further solutions have to be considered in order to address this problem.

The Soviet model of ambulance response only transports about 50% to 60% of all patients as many patients are treated by physician-lead teams that spend significant time on scene (unpublished data, Osh Ambulance Service, & own observations). The reasons for not-transport decisions are plenty: Hospitals have only a limited number of beds & supplies. The cardiology unit will not accept any patients that are not having ECG evidence of an acute myocardial infarction. Ambulance doctors act as gatekeepers and restrict care. Many examples could show frequent observations which show patients suffering from hypertensive crisis or angina pectoris are left at home after an initial treatment and that hospitals refuse to accept patients if the ambulance team can not present a ECG (electro cardiogram) printout with signs of a fresh myocardial infarction.

All acute calls were selected for data analysis on ambulance response times. This resulted in 260 acute calls in the first week of data collection and 249 acute calls in the second week of data collection. Cardiovascular emergencies with an average of 30% were the majority of all cases in the first and the second week. Other types of acute cases were recorded less often (Table-5).

The World Health Organization European Office has published data that shows that three causes for early mortality in the Kyrgyz Republic (McKee, 2002) are (1.) cardiovascular diseases, (2.) cancer, and (3.) injuries. The data also points out that cardiovascular diseases are 5 times higher in the Kyrgyz Republic than in Europe. On the other hand the data reveals that only 21 of 509 ambulance response cases are related to trauma (Table-5). This number is even more surprising as trauma is seen as one of the three major disease groups in the Kyrgyz Republic. Trauma especially includes in Kyrgyzstan: road traffic accidents, domestic violence due to alcoholism, drowning and burn injuries. For this reason it is interesting to note that there are only a few ambulance response cases that are of a trauma nature. The data confirms a study by Ibrahimov (2002). He found that mostly all trauma patients get immediate transportation by taxi or private car to the reception unit of the Osh City Hospital or the Osh Regional Hospital. This data shows that the ambulance service is bypassed and only in a few cases is asked to respond to trauma incidents. It can be said that the ambulance service is not utilized for trauma care as the population is not informed about the nature of trauma and the ambulance service has a long response time. This contributes to the high level of injury and morbidity in these trauma cases.

Behavior like this is typical for the region and the cultural background of the population. Similar behavior in trauma cases was noticed in Karachi, Pakistan as well as in Dhaka, Bangladesh. The authors of these papers conclude that the reason for this behavior is lack of accessibility, cultural barriers and lack of education in order to recognize danger sings (Razzak, 2001; Andersson, 1998). Poor ambulance response performance in trauma cases might trigger the population to rather organize transportation of patients themselves than to rely on the ambulance service. In order to change this behavior for the benefit of patients suffering from a health emergency first aid education should be reinforced.

A poor response time might also be the reason why several callers have called a second and a third time in order to enquire the situation about the ambulance responding. In the first week data recording there where 507 calls recorded and categorized (Table 3). In this first week 260 acute conditions, 66 patient advices and 33 re-calls by patients where recorded (Table-5). 4 patients even called a third time (Table-3) In the second week data recording there where 416 calls, 249 were urgent, 64 were patient advice, 19 callers had to call a second time and 2 callers called even a third time (Table-3). The reason for some callers to call a second and a third time might be that the ambulance time is perceived as being to long.

6. Conclusion

A search of the literature has shown that the development of emergency health care systems in developing countries is of increasing importance. Osh in the southern part of Kyrgyzstan has been chosen as an example for a developing urban emergency health care system. Emergency medical dispatch training has been chosen as an important organizational instrument to improve EMS performance. Ambulance response time as an indicator for emergency medical service performance has been identified. There is an increasing interest in low-cost but effective measurements to improve emergency health care. Therefore the question was if dispatcher training can improve ambulance response times in EMS systems in low income countries.

The study has shown that implementing low-cost changes like a specifically tailored emergency medical dispatch program and technical changes in dispatching ambulance crews can likely improve ambulance response times. The observed time improvement will probably have only a limited impact on patients' health status and the overall system performance as other factors also contribute to relatively slow ambulance response time. Some factors could be controlled by the ambulance service (organization, human resources); others need a more widespread intervention in order to improve the overall outcome.

Some authors have questioned the approach in emergency health care development to look only for a single indicator like ambulance response time to measure the performance of an emergency medical service system. However if a case sensitive approach is chosen and a particular system is carefully evaluated ambulance response time can become a major indicator for the overall system performance. Further research of other subjects with a focus on emergency medical dispatch and emergency medical response in the developing world could bring further clarity. Health care priorities and the pressing needs to invest in the development of emergency health care systems in resource-limited countries support this demand. The need for further research will likely increase as more low- and middle- income countries recognize the need for improved emergency health care in their countries (Jamison (Ed.), 2006).

Worldwide mobility, information technology and further globalization increase opportunities for emergency health care professionals to play an increasing role in supporting research and development of emergency medical services in less developed regions of the world for the benefit of its populations.

References

Andersson, R., & Rahman, F., & Svanström, L. (1998). Medical help seeking behaviour of injury patients in a community in Bangladesh. Public Health 112, 31-35.

Arreola-Risa, C., & Carazos, L., & Jorkovich G. J., & Maier R.V., & Mock, C.N., & Padilla, P. (1995, September). Trauma care systems in urban Latin America: The priorities should be prehospital and ER management. Journal of Trauma: Injury, Infection and Critical Care 30.3, 457-462.

Arreola-Risa, C., & Canavati-Ayub, F., & de la Cruz, O., & Garcia, C., & Jurkovich, G. J., & Mock, C. N., & Losero-Wheatly, L. (2000). Low-cost improvements in prehospital trauma care in a Latin American city. The Journal of Trauma: Injury, Infection and Critical Care 48(1), 119-124.

Brown, L.H., & Whitney, C.L., & Addario, M., & Hogue, T., & Hunt, R.C., (2000, January March). Do warning lights and sirens reduce ambulance response times? Prehospital Emergency Care 4(1), 70-74.

Davis, M. A. (2004). Emergency medicine and international health: Increasing impact by broadening the mandate. Annals of Emergency Medicine 43, e9-e10.

Farlane, M., & Been, C.A. (2003) Evaluation of emergency medical services systems: A classification to assist in determination of indicators. Emergency Medical Journal 20, 188-191.

Finch, H., & Gerard, W.C., & Harvey, A.L., & Riece, G.F. Jr. (1999, January-March). Actual vs. perceived EMS response time. Prehospital Emergency Care 3(1), 11-14.

Hauswald, M., & Yeoh, E. (1997, October). Designing a prehospital system for a developing country: estimated cost and benefits. American Journal of Emergency Medicine 15(6), 600-603.

Ibrahimov, S. (2002). Self-referral patterns of patients seeking care from either the ambulance service or family medicine-related institutions in Osh. - Osh emergency care research project. Bishkek: Scientific Technology & Language Institute Inc.

Jamison, D. T., & Breman, J.G., & Mesham, R., & Alleyne, G., & Claeson, M., & Evans, D.B., & Mills, A., & Musgrove, P. A., & Sha, P. (Ed.). (2006). Disease control priorities in developing countries – 2nd edition. Oxford: Oxford University Press, World Bank, 1261-1280.

Kellermann, A.L., & Razzak, J. A. (2002). Emergency medical care in developing countries: is it worthwhile? Bulletin of the World Health Organization 80(11), 900-905.

Kobusingye, O. C., & Hyder, A. A., & Bishai, D., & Hicks, E. R., & Joshipura, M.& Mock, C. (2005, August). Emergency medical systems in low- and middle- income countries: recommendations for action. Bulletin of the World Health Organization 83(8), 626-631.

Mayer, J.D. (1979, August). Emergency medical service: delays, response time and survival. Medical Care 17(8), 818-827.

McKee, M., & Healy, J., & Falkingham, J. (Ed.). (2002). Health care in Central Asia – European observatory on health care systems. Buckingham: Open University Press & World Health Organization.

McSwain, N. E. (1991). Prehospital emergency medical systems and cardiopulmonary resuscitation – Trauma 2nd edition. Norwalk, CT: Appleton and Lange, 99-107

Meimanaliev, A.S., & Ibrahimova, A., & Elebesov, B., & Rechel, B. (2005). Healthcare systems in transition: Kyrgyzstan. Copenhagen: WHO Regional Office for Europe on behalf of the European Observatory on Health Systems and Policies, 2005.

Mock, C., & Arreola-Risa, C., & Quanash, R. (2003, April). Strengthening care for injured persons in less developed countries: A case study of Ghana and Mexico. Injury Prevention and Safety Promotion 10(1-2), 45-51.

Mock, C.N., & Jurkovich, G.S., & nii-Amon-Kotei, D., & Arreola-Risa, C., & Maier, R.V. (1998). Trauma mortality patterns in three nations at different economic levels: implications for global trauma systems development. Journal of Trauma 44, 804-812.

Moore, L. (1999, October-December). Measuring quality and effectiveness of prehospital EMS. Prehospital Emergency Care 3(4), 325-331.

O'Meara, P. (2005). A generic performance framework for ambulance services: an Australian health services perspective. Journal of Emergency Primary Health Care 3(3), 1-13.

Partridge, R.A. (1998, October). Emergency medicine in West Kazakhstan, CIS. <u>Annals of Emergency Medicine 32</u>(4), 493-497.

Payne, D. (2000, November 11). Poor ambulance response causes 700 deaths annually in Ireland. <u>British Medical Journal 321,</u> 1176.

Pell, P. J., & Coble, S.M., & Ford, I., & Marsden, A.K., & Sivel, M.J. (2001, June 9). Effect of reducing ambulance response times on death from out of hospital cardiac arrest: a cohort study. <u>British Medical Journal 322,</u> 1385-1388.

Pozner, C.N., & Bayleygne, T.M., & Davis, M.A., & Benin, G., & Halpen, P., & Noble, V.E. (2003, July-September). Emergency medical services capacities in the developing world: preliminary evaluation and training in Addis Ababa, Ethiopia. <u>Prehospital Emergency Care 7</u>(3), 392-396.

Razzak, J.A., & Cone, D.C., & Rehmani, R. (2001, July-September). Emergency medical services and cultural determinants of an emergency in Karachi, Pakistan. <u>Prehospital Emergency Care 5</u>(3), 312-316.

Shepard, H. (1999, May). <u>Emergency medicine in Bishkek, Kyrgyzstan.</u> Bishkek: Scientific Technology & Language Institute Inc.

Stiell, I.G., & Campeau, T., & Dagnone, E., & De Mario, V.J., & Field, B.J., & Lunistra, L.G., & Lyver, M.B., & Maloney, J., & Munkley, D.P., & Spaite, D.W., & Ward, R., & Wells,

G.A. (1999, September 15). Improvement in out-of-hospital cardiac arrest survival through the

inexpensive optimization of an existing defibrillation program: OPALS study phase II. Ontario

Prehospital Advanced Life Support. JAMA 282(11), 1033-1034.

Townes, D.A., & Gulo, S., & Lee, T. E., & Van Rooyen, M. J., (1998, August).

Emergency medicine in Russia. Annals of Emergency Medicine 32(2), 239-242.

Wallace, D., & Anderson, M., & Luneke, L. (Ed.). (1995). National highway traffic safety

administration – Emergency medical dispatch: national standard curriculum – Instructor's guide.

Washington: The Learning Group Cooperation, National Highway Traffic Safety Administration.

Appendix

Graph-1   Difference in response times from the first to the second week of data collection
before and after training.

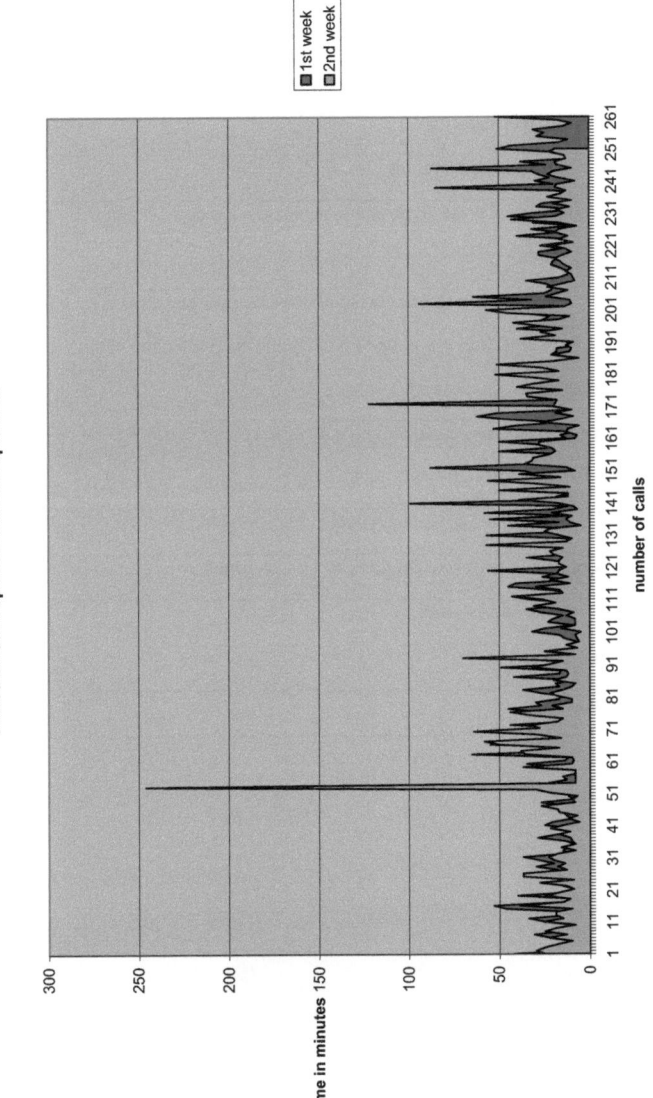

Table – 1   Elements of the research design

Research Design
• Development of Data Collection Form
• Information on the Research Project of all participating institutions (Osh Ambulance Service, Osh EMS Training Center).
• Selection of Research Assistant
• Data collection First Week (6 days in one week, each day 7 hours, 3 days morning hours, 3 days evening hours)
• Development of training course based on the US EMD curricula from 1995, including text, handouts, guide booklet and power point presentations. Translation of the whole material into Russian language
• Training of 6 feldsher-dispatchers on a 40 hour course (5 days) DPS-program (based on USDOT- EMD curriculum)
• Informal training of the ambulance staff in early morning briefings
• Implementation of technical changes at the Osh Ambulance Station
• Data collection second week
• Processing of data
• Analysis of data

Table-2   Elements of the audio visual address and activation system.

Audio/Visual address and activation system
• Flashing light / speaker combination in each room of the ambulance station.
• Flashing light / speaker combination for the ambulance station yard and parking lot for ambulance vehicles.
• Technical changes in FM radio system in order to transmit additional audio signal for urgent calls.
• Technical changes at the dispatch center in order to transmit audio/visual signals in order to activate ambulance crews for urgent calls.

Table- 3   Calls recorded as to call type and classified when applicable as to preliminary diagnosis by the dispatcher both before and after training

call type	week 1 data number	week 2 data number
abdominal pain	10	21
coronary condition	26	28
psychotic condition	12	6
airway obstruction	1	0
allergic reaction	6	4
asked address	11	7
anemia	0	1
asked # of hospital	0	1
animal bite	1	0
asthma attack	8	3
back pain	1	2
bad patient condition	2	23
bleeding	5	1
high blood pressure	55	46
burn injuries	0	2
caller called 2nd time	29	18
caller called 3rd time	4	3
chronic pain	1	0
diarrhea	1	1
influenza	4	0
fracture (open)	1	4
high temperature	26	20
headache	4	4
head trauma	3	2
hepatitis	0	1
homicide	3	0
kidney pain	1	2
laceration	0	2
labor pain (premature)	2	3
menstrual problems	1	0
lung edema	0	1
misplaced call	93	41
needs injection	0	1
nosebleed	0	1
phone advice	66	64
pneumonia	0	1
poisoning	4	3
private call	44	33
seizures	7	6
feels sick	3	6
stroke	5	3
transfer	4	11*
trauma	8	0
Urologic problem	0	1
Unconscious patient	40	17
Unknown patient condition	12	16
vomiting	3	4
		2
total	507	416

* transfer including two pregnant patients

Table-4   Acute calls analyzed as to type

	Week 1 data	Week 1 data	Week 2 data	Week 2 data
	number	percentage	number	percentage
Cardiovascular System	81	31.2	74	29.7
Trauma	13	5.0	8	3.2
Unconscious	40	15.4	17	6.8
Other	112	43.1	109	43.8
unknown	14	5.4	41	16.5
total	**260**		**249**	

Table-5   All calls analyzed as to type

	Week 1 data number	Week 1 data percentage	Week 2 data number	Week 2 data percentage
acute conditions	260	51.3	249	59.9
private calls	44	8.7	33	7.9
patient advice	66	13.0	64	15.4
re calls by patient	33	6.5	21	5.0
asked address	11	2.2	8	1.9
misplaced calls	93	18.3	41	9.9
total	507		416	

Table – 6   Average response time before (week1) and after (week2) intervention, including
standard deviation and t-value.

	Average response time in minutes	Standard deviation in minutes	t-value
Before intervention (week 1)	23,09	17,67	1,647847
After intervention (week 2)	20,15	18,43	1,647847